How To

A How To Ta[lk Dirty] That Will Make Your Partner Beg For You! + 10 Great Examples

Jennifer Amor

Table of Contents

Introduction 3

Chapter 1: The Language of Lust 6

Chapter 2: The Nice Thing About Being Naughty 13

Chapter 3: Working on Your Carnal Candor 21

Chapter 4: Mastering the Art of Erotic Eloquence 34

Chapter 5: The Don'ts of Dirty Talk 40

Chapter 6: Filthy Fun - Examples of Sexy Phrases to Leave Your Lover Begging for More 44

Conclusion 49

Introduction

I want to thank you and congratulate you for purchasing the book, "**How To Talk Dirty**"

This book contains proven steps and strategies on how to use the language of lust to drive your lover mad with carnal desire.

There are thousands of books that talk about giving and receiving pleasure through the genitals and the erogenous zones. Even so, they neglect to pay attention to the most important sex organ that humans possess: the brain. Within the brain is a limitless reserve of sensual stimuli. Uttering the right words can heighten one's state of arousal and even enhance the intensity of orgasms.

Dirty words have the power to connect you with your primal nature. It helps couples strip away inhibitions and to unleash the wild lovers within. But more importantly, titillating talk enables you to delve into your significant other's mind. It encourages your partner to share with you his/her raw thoughts and emotions thus, making sex infinitely more intimate. Now, if only you could get over the awkwardness and fear of rejection…

Through this book, you will learn what dirty talk is and how it can benefit your sex life and your relationship. More than that, you will learn how to talk dirty without feeling like an ass. Find out about the rules of talking dirty and how to correctly introduce titillating talk into your lovemaking routine. In a manner of speaking, this book will teach you how to fuck your lover's brains out.

Filthy words put the fun in fucking. But how dirty is too dirty? This book also discusses the don'ts of dirty talk. In the last chapter, you'll find ten great examples of sexy sentences that will keep your sexual soulmate begging for more.

Read on. This is your ultimate guide to erotic eloquence.

Thanks again for purchasing this book, I hope you enjoy it!

Chapter 1: The Language of Lust

What is dirty talk?

Dirty talk, in the simplest sense, refers to sex play which involves sensual phrasing with the purpose of igniting your partner's desire. Naughty language works by triggering one's imagination thus, building your lover's arousal before and during intercourse. Dirty talk does its job by stimulating your sexual soulmate's bodily senses (sound, touch, sight, etc.) by triggering his/her brain and thus, inducing a desired response.

Couples use dirty talk as a means of expressing what they want and need from their partner while they're caught up in the heat of passionate lovemaking.

What are the types of dirty talk?

<u>Soft Core</u>

This is also known as "sweet nothings". The language used in soft core dirty talking is not dirty per se. Rather, they are meant to sound warm, encouraging, and even affectionate. The purpose of soft core dirty talk is to appeal to your lover's emotions and to draw a response from his/her feelings of affection towards you.

Soft core dirty talk is a great way to introduce hardcore love lingo into the bedroom. Use it as a means to prepare your partner, to get a sense of his feelings about sexy talk, and to gauge his boundaries.

Examples:

"You're the hottest thing I've ever seen."

"I want to hold you so badly."

"I love the stuff that you do with your fingers."

"Baby, I've never felt so good."

These phrases may seem terribly lukewarm. That said, the secret to making soft core phrases sound utterly dirty is by controlling *how you say it*. It all depends on how you want your lover to feel and what response you wish to get out of him/her. If you want your message to come across as passionate and aggressive, say it with a gruff voice or through gritted teeth, like you're struggling to stop yourself from ravaging your lover. If you want to sound romantic and adoring, assume a soft tone and say it with a sigh.

Another factor that greatly affects the meaning behind your message is the direction of your gaze. A soft core phrase like "You're the hottest thing I've ever seen." can easily turn into hard core dirty talk when you're looking at your lover's genitals rather than his/her face.

Likewise, the context has the capacity to influence the definition of your words. For instance, when a man says "Baby, I've never felt so good", it holds a more hardcore meaning when the couple is in the midst of intercourse and he's deep inside the woman. The exact same words tend to be softer core when he says it in the midst of lip-lock during foreplay. Again, the very same words will have a different meaning when he utters it after intercourse and while he and his woman are cuddling. In this case, the words "Baby, I've never felt so good." turns from stimulating to reassuring.

Hardcore

As opposed to soft core dirty talking, hardcore phrases tend to be more direct and at most times, seemingly vulgar. The purpose is to yield a physical response rather than an emotional one. Hardcore dirty talk appeals to the primal instinct... the animalistic nature, if you will. They encourage even the most modest individuals to unleash the beast within. Hardcore words urge a person to drop their inhibitions at the bedroom doorstep, to feel free to give in to pleasure, and to be at liberty to express themselves.

During hardcore dirty talking, swear words may be included. One might ask: *How does profanity suddenly become sexy?* When you don't usually use swearwords and then end up blurting them out during lovemaking, it gives the impression of losing control. It makes your lover feel that the sex is so good that you scarcely know how to describe it, and thus, you resort to using coarse language.

Couples often use hardcore words as a means to push boundaries as well as to make sexual role play seem more realistic. We all play various roles in real life (ex. the doting mom, the good wife, the kind neighbor, the disciplined employee, etc.) and all of these characters are bound by rules of proper behavior. By saying words which you don't typically use while playing these characters, you enable yourself to strip off all those roles and just feel free to become a sensual being with a boundless capacity to give and receive pleasure.

Hardcore talk also serves as a secret shared between couples and for this reason, it deepens your intimacy. The beauty of hardcore sex lingo is that it comes off as raw and honest. The sheer bluntness of it all shows your partner that the words spring from deep within you. Simply put, hardcore dirty talk makes your partner feel that he/she has accessed a side of you which you rarely reveal.

Examples:

"I'm hungry, honey. Sit on my face."

"I want you to cum in my throat."

"Oh, baby... Those tits are made for fucking."

"Oh yes! *This* is what a real man's cock feels like!"

Cock... Pussy... Cunt... Fuck... Tits... *Must I really use this kind of language?* Well, you don't have to if you don't want to. The key to successful dirty talk is to use words that you and your partner are comfortable with.

Some women may find the word "cunt" offensive. Meanwhile, some women may find colorful euphemisms like "blossom" or "jewel" downright corny and hence, extremely unsexy.

Take a look at these sentences and examine how you feel:

"I want to lick your pussy."

"I want to lick your vagina."

"I want to lick your flower."

Some men, often married ones with kids, may find the word "vagina" a tad too clinical. It may conjure images of slack, overstretched lips and infants pushing their way out of their mothers' hooch. Imagine licking *that*.

In the end, the key is to observe your partner's reaction or better yet, ask him/her how he/she feels about each naughty word. Come up with a list of modern sex jargons and discuss it with your partner. Make it a fun activity. Highlight the hot ones and laugh at the ridiculous ones. In the succeeding chapters, we'll discuss ways on how to get your erotic phraseology right.

Chapter 2: The Nice Thing About Being Naughty

How can dirty talk improve my sex life and my relationships?

First, let's talk about the most obvious benefit: **dirty talk makes sex several degrees hotter.**

The number one secret to successful sex is open communication. The ego is a fragile thing. One of the worst things that could happen during sex is when you utter a suggestion and then it gets misconstrued. Dirty talk gives you and your lover a means to express your wants and needs and to give feedback in a totally non-offensive way.

Take a look at this comment:

Woman: "Don't come yet. This time, let me go first."

Honest? Yes.

Informative? Yup.

Helpful? Not so much.

Sexy? Definitely not.

Though the woman's intention is good, this sentence is likely to make a man feel as though:

- a) she's accusing him of being selfish
- b) she's criticizing his style
- c) she's telling him how to make love and thus, she thinks that he doesn't know what he's doing
- d) she's not even close to climaxing and so all his hard work has come to nothing.

Here's a fact: Any words uttered during sex can be a distraction from pleasure so when you say something during intercourse, *make sure that it's worth it.*

Now, take a look at the "naughtified" version of this feedback:

"Oh, baby, keep doing that and I'm gonna come really soon..."

See the difference? Giving instructions while doing the deed may distract one's partner, dampen the mood, and discourage him /her. But if you tweak your words a bit and turn them into sexy talk, they end up motivating your partner to perform better in the sack.

When you are able to tell your lover what to do and where and when and how you want it, all without wounding his ego, how can that possibly not lead to great sex?

Dirty talk boosts your partner's confidence in bed.

Dirty talk has the power to turn so-so lovers into alpha males and shy women into carnal goddesses. If you want great sex, then make it your business to build your lover's ego. Women who are overly self-conscious about their bodies are unlikely to agree to bold bedroom ideas like doing a striptease or trying sex positions that make them feel too exposed.

Positive body image is vital for great sex. When a person looks at his/her reflection in the mirror and sees someone undesirable, the idea works its way into his subconscious so that it automatically lowers the person's libido. Thus, no matter how attractive his partner is, one remains difficult to arouse.

Simply put, in order to be turned on by your partner, you first need to be turned on by yourself.

Men may experience performance anxiety and worry about premature ejaculation, their staying power, the size of their penis, etc. Some men may seem confident on the outside but in fact, they feel threatened about the idea of relinquishing control in the bedroom. Hence, they may be afraid of being handcuffed or they may feel nervous about having their nipples touched.

Use dirty talk to assure your man of his prowess in bed or to compliment your woman's gorgeous body.

Example:

"I love running my tongue over your curves."

"It's beautiful the way your breasts bounce when you move on top of me."

"I love how your cock fills me."

It keeps you and your partner in tune with each other.

Another nice thing about naughty talk between the sheets is that it encourages lovers to become more verbal instead of leaving their partner to guess several things like what they're feeling, what they're thinking, or where the clit is located. Moaning, sighing, and screaming are all wonderful but the trouble is they can easily be misinterpreted.

Take a look at this typical scenario:

Girl screams out of pleasure. Worried, guy stops what he's doing and asks her: "Did I hurt you?"

Frustrating isn't it?

It would've been better if she had used dirty talk to tell her man that he was on the right track. Something as simple as: "Don't stop, baby. It feels so good." would have done the trick.

Erotic lingo gets the creative juices *and* the love juices flowing.

It's never a good thing for couples when things get boring between the sheets. The thing about naughty talk is that it awakens an adventurous, creative, and deeply sensual side of you. It's a fact that words easily become actions. Perhaps now your erotic vocab may be limited to "Oh God, I'm coming." but in no time, you'll be saying things like "I'm going to drop by your office, shut the blinds, tie you up in your chair, and lick you 'til you beg me to fuck you."

When you say these words out loud, they are implanted into your subconscious and into that of your lover's. You build up this fantasy scenario and it will keep playing itself up in your mind. Pretty soon, you'll be paying him/her a visit at work with a pair of handcuffs in your pocket.

Naughty talk is fantastic foreplay *and* afterplay.

Dirty talk is not just done during lovemaking but also before and after sex. Compared to men, it takes longer for women to get sexually aroused. Dirty talk, be it soft core or hardcore, can play a vital role in helping a woman get in the mood for love. Men enjoy being teased just as much. The thing about orgasms is that the longer the anticipation and the more powerful the build-up, the stronger and the more pleasurable they become. So whisper some sexy words while you're taking each other's clothes off. Do a little sexting to build your lover's excitement.

If there's one thing that men love more than ejaculating, it's knowing that they were able to satisfy their women. Likewise, women want to be reassured of their lover's affection and satisfaction after lovemaking. After having sex, use dirty talk as a means to communicate your joy and gratitude.

Example:

"I love that little thing that you did with your tongue."

"I don't think anyone can make me come as hard as you can."

When done correctly, this may even motivate your lover to go for another round.

Chapter 3: Working on Your Carnal Candor

How do I talk dirty without feeling like a fool?

The thing about dirty talk is that it can be quite challenging even to the most verbose people. Some words may come across as sexy on paper but when said out loud, they might sound absolutely ridiculous. Even those who are completely confident in the sack might think: "OMG, I can't imagine myself saying that." After all, for most couples, sex has always been about action. So how does one get the words to fit in? Furthermore, how do you stop yourself from feeling like a total idiot?

First, work with yourself.

It's normal to feel weird at first about talking dirty during sex, especially if you're not used to vulgar vocabulary. Try masturbating and while you're doing it, talk dirty to yourself. Imagine that you're making love with your partner. What do you want to say to him/her? Describe the sensations that you're experiencing while you're pleasuring yourself and try to find the exact words to describe them. You may begin by talking dirty in your head and then eventually start speaking it out loud.

Develop a positive outlook.

V-v-vagina... There are some people who are uncomfortable with their sexual organs being the subject of any conversation. However, you need to understand that mentioning one's genitals is not dirty in itself. Stand naked in front of the mirror and look at your body. If you're a woman, take a mirror down there and spread your legs wide open. Touch your body parts and say their names out loud. Observe them and describe what you love most about them.

Example:

Touch your breasts and say: "My boobs are full and beautiful. I love how pink my nipples are."

Always concentrate on the positive. If your penis is short, then focus on how easily it fills with blood and how quickly it gets hard and ready for action. If you have thick thighs, refer to them as your thunder thighs.

Before you are able to appreciate your partner's body, you must first be able to appreciate your own.

Develop an open mind.

Understand that it's all sex play. Dirty talk does not cheapen you, your partner, or the relationship. Talking dirty is not about disrespecting your lover or devaluing the act of lovemaking. Some women may love being called a bitch, a slut, or a whore in the sack but that doesn't mean that they want to be treated that way, especially out of the bedroom. Likewise, a man may love being called a slave behind closed doors but that doesn't mean that he has a weak character.

Enrich your erotic vocab.

There are a hundred words that you can use to refer to sex and to your genitals. Therefore, there shouldn't be any reason not to find one that does not offend you or your partner. Search for current sex slangs on the internet, read erotica, and watch sensual artistic films with your hubby/wifey. Then together, determine which words work for the both of you.

Look at these alternative names for fucking and examine how you feel about them:

Boning

Bumping uglies

Shagging

Bonking

Nookie

Getting it on

Screwing

The lust and thrust

Bump and grind

Which of these would you use?

Other names for the vagina:

Honey pot

Fanny

Kitty

Vag

Pussy

Cunt

Snatch

Beaver

Juicebox

Poonany

Bikini bizkit

Cherry pop

Honeysuckle

Passion fruit

Jewel box

Altar of Venus

If you want to describe the pussy, how many positive adjectives do you have up your sleeve?

Juicy

Succulent

Yummy

Moist

Luscious

Mouthwatering

Explore these other terms for the penis:

Cock

Dick

Trouser snake

Pole

Joystick

Cum gun

Dipstick

Dragon

Fuck rod

Love rod

Jackhammer

Love muscle

Which of these turn you on? Which words are funny? Which ones are offensive?

How many words can you comfortably use to describe your orgasm to your partner?

Out-of-this-world

Amazing

Fantastic

Cosmic

Earth-shattering

Bone-shaking

Incredible

Soul-moving

Magical

Spine-shivering

Otherworldly

Crazed

You don't have to be a verbal gymnast to please your partner but dirty talk can quickly turn stale when you run out of synonyms for "good" and "hot".

Talk about sex.

Introducing dirty talk into the relationship becomes easier when you and your significant other are able to discuss sex openly with each other. After making love, make it a point to talk about how you felt, the love moves that you enjoyed, the things that you want him/her to do again, etc. The more specific you are, the better.

Example: "It felt really good when you slipped a finger up my ass while I was coming. I'd love it if you do it again next time."

Find out how your lover feels about dirty talk. Break it to him/her gently. For instance, watch together a film with lots of racy talk. Then, later, ask your lover how he/she feels about it.

Turn your bedroom into a judgment-free zone.

One of the greatest obstacles for introducing dirty talk in the bedroom is when one is afraid of being rejected by his/her lover. When your partner suggests something, fight your initial urge to laugh or to burst out indignations. Instead, listen with an open mind and an open heart. While in the midst of making love and your lover says something that you don't particularly like, don't reprimand your partner on the spot. Instead, talk about it later.

Example:

"I want to talk to you about when you called me a little whore earlier. I'm down with the "whore" part. But maybe next time, we can drop the "little"?

Establish ground rules together and respect them.

To prevent dirty talk from being just plain filthy, establish your rules. Negotiate about the words that you're willing and not willing to use.

Example:

"You can call me a slut but I don't think I'm ready to be called a cockwash."

Start with dirty writing.

Begin by sending each other naughty texts or emails. Writing down sexy words is less embarrassing than telling it to someone face-to-face. You can start with a brief note.

Ex: "I keep thinking about making love to you."

Then, you may progress to racier texts.

Ex: "Such a shame you're not around. Now I'm going to have to touch myself."

Start with simple sexy phrases.

Unless it's used to hit the G-spot, pressure can be bad for sex. So, start slow. Begin by paying attention to what your lover is doing to you and then describe how it makes you feel.

Example:

"Your tongue feels so good on my nipples."

Experiment with various voices to find your own.

Are you a screaming goddess or a sighing flower? A roaring animal or a grunting beast? Experiment from high-pitched howling to clear whispers. This way, you might even get to unveil a previously undiscovered side of your personality. Make yourself unpredictable. Dirty talk can get dull when your lover can tell exactly when you're going to open your mouth. One of the most powerful tricks in naughty talk is catching your partner unaware.

Dirty dialogue is a two-way street.

It's necessary to prevent a more loquacious lover from dominating the dirty talk. As a matter of fact, it would be good to urge the quieter person to speak up more during lovemaking. Use it as a means to learn more about your partner. Generally, couples must take turns with being on the giving end and on the receiving end. By being able to experience the roles of a talker and a listener, you're able develop a balanced perspective. Everything about good sex is a result of successful give and take.

Make your own love lingo.

Just because "driving up the Hershey Highway" is a modern slang for anal sex, that doesn't mean that you have to use it. Especially, if it makes you think of feces. Naughty talk is meant to titillate, not to disgust. If you feel that the current coital colloquial does nothing to stir your desire, feel free to invent your own language of lust. Sharing a secret language which only the two of you understand is another way to deepen your intimacy with your partner.

Example:

"Let's invent another name for "finger blasting". The word makes it sound rather painful."

Chapter 4: Mastering the Art of Erotic Eloquence

What can I do to develop my skills in dirty talking?

The Past, the Present, and the Future

The easiest way to perform dirty talk is to talk about what you're doing, what you're going to do, and finally, about what you did.

Tell your lover what you want to do to him/her.

Example:

While dining at a restaurant, lean over and whisper these words to his/her ear: "I want to go down the table and eat your cock/pussy for dinner."

Do it.

You don't necessarily have to give your partner oral in public but nothing's more terrible than an empty promise. So, give your partner a little downtown loving' as soon as you get him/her alone.

While fulfilling your promise, say something like: "Mmm… You taste so good. This was all I could think about at dinner."

If you're the receiving party, be sure to reciprocate. Nothing's more awkward than listening to a soliloquy about your genitals during lovemaking.

Prolong your lover's pleasure by using dirty talk even after sex.

When you're done, say something like: "I love how you filled my mouth with your love juice." This will trigger your sexual soulmate to respond. Your lover is likely to say what he/she would like to do to you in return.

<u>Handle awkward dirty talk with tact.</u>

What do you do when the dirty talk is starting to make you feel uncomfortable? How do you get an overly talkative lover to shut up? Try to make your scolding sound sexy.

Example:

"Shut up and suck me."

"I don't want you to talk dirty, baby. I want you to *play* dirty."

Be natural.

Nothing can kill desire faster than a fake compliment. Unfortunately, it's easy to be superfluous when you're really just trying to sound sexy and spontaneous. Here's a helpful tip: Just say what's on your mind. If you think her pussy is wonderfully tight, just say it. You don't need to spout pussy poetry just to let her know that it feels great to be inside her. The important thing is that you mean what you say and that your lover knows it.

While it's alright to assume a different role during lovemaking, it is necessary to incorporate something of yourself into that role. This way, your lover will still feel that he/she is making love with you instead of with a total stranger. Remember that successful sex and relationships are based on honesty and trust.

Timing is everything.

A sexy word dropped at the wrong moment can interfere with mounting desire. Wait for your lover to get sufficiently heated before you progress into hardcore lust lingo. In other words, lube up before you stick it up the ass. You'll find that it's easier to drop naughty suggestions after a round of passionate kissing or fondling.

Find out what your lover's trigger words are.

Trigger words refer to terms that once heard by your lover, have the capacity to turn them into untamed beasts. The easiest way to do this is to let your lover do the talking. Ask your partner what he/she wants you to do to him/her.

Example: "Tell me how you want me to touch you."

Your significant other will respond with words which he/she finds most sensual.

Sometimes, all it takes is one word.

Dirty talk doesn't have to be lengthy. Often, single words like "Yes", "More", and "Harder" can sufficiently do the trick. During lovemaking, you may substitute some of your moans and grunts with these one-word directives.

Concentrate on the physical aspect.

The great thing about dirty talk is that it encourages mindful sex. It enables you to actually be in the present and to direct your attention to what is actually happening between the sheets. Define how your lover makes you feel before you verbalize it. Focus on the feeling of the cock sliding in and out and then describe it. Use definite words like hot, hard, warm, wet, pulsating, etc. What does your lover's skin smell like? What does your partner's lips taste like? Engage all of your senses.

Chapter 5: The Don'ts of Dirty Talk

What common mistakes must I avoid when talking dirty?

<u>Don't fixate too much on size.</u>

Whether it's the penis or the breasts or the vagina or the thighs, don't comment too much on bodily proportions. This can easily be misunderstood. Moreover, you might end up hitting your lover's insecurities without meaning to. You may think that your lady love's small breasts are awesome but she might hate it when you make her feel like a boob less wonder. Likewise, refrain from calling a man's cock "humongous" when you both know he's just average. A better alternative would be to praise his rock hard erection or to notice her sensitive nipples.

<u>Don't say it unless you intend to deliver the goods.</u>

If you say things like "You've been a naughty girl/boy. I'm going to punish you.", then make sure that you do. More importantly, make sure that your partner knows that you intend to follow through with your words. Otherwise, all that dirty talk loses its impact.

Be careful about planting seeds of false hope into your lover's head. Unless you're actually willing to explore a new kind of kink, don't even hint at the possibility.

Don't force yourself to say stuff just to please your lover.

If you do, it will inevitably show. As mentioned in the previous chapter, it is necessary to set dirty talking rules with your partner. This is to ensure that the both of you get pleasure out of it.

Don't memorize sexy phrases.

It's better to come up with your own lines than to Google a bunch of naughty words made by others. There's nothing less sexy than a rehearsed atmosphere. Remember, there's no other person in this world who understands what makes your sexual soulmate tick.

Don't use dirty talk as a way to fish for compliments.

That's unless you're open to the possibility of disappointment. When you ask your lover questions like: "Did you like what I did with my mouth?", you are asking it for him/her and not to feed your own ego. Additionally, fishing for compliments shows a lack of confidence which is extremely unattractive.

Don't slip into vagueness or vulgarity.

Saying stuff like "Oh yeah, that feels good." tends to get old quickly. It comes across as lazy and mechanical and even insincere. As previously mentioned, you need to be more specific and more descriptive. Pay real attention to what your partner is doing. They'll love you all the more for it.

Example: "That twirling trick that you did with your tongue around my shaft... That was incredible."

Dirty talk like "Oh yeah, fuck my tight pussy!" reeks of poorly directed porn. When you copy dirty language from pornography, it's like you're insulting your lover's intelligence. The last thing that you want your sexual soulmate to think is that you're faking it for him/her. It wounds his/her ego instead of boosting it. Your lover will end up doubting his/her skills. Which leads us to our next don't…

Don't ever attempt to pull off a fake orgasm.

Once you do, your lover will wonder whether all those other explosive orgasms he/she had given you in the past are all just phony.

As hot as it may sound, don't tell your lover stuff like "You make me so hard/wet." unless it's true because… well, they can tell when you're lying.

Don't forget to laugh.

Too much tension can leave you tongue-tied. Couples in successful relationships understand the value of laughing *with* each other rather than *at* each other. Expect a few bumps along the road, and use good humor to deal with the blunders.

Chapter 6: Filthy Fun - Examples of Sexy Phrases to Leave Your Lover Begging for More

Naughty words to say to your woman:

"I love the way your ____ looks/smells/tastes/feels like _____."

Ex: "I love the way your skin tastes like vanilla. It makes me want to lick you over and over."

To turn a shy flower into an erotic queen, you need to boost her self-confidence. It's not enough to tell her that she's beautiful or that she's hot. After all, she probably hears that all the time. Highlight her specific qualities that excite you.

Another way to do this is when you're not in the midst of having sex and when you're both completely clothed. This way, there is less chance of accidentally touching on any of her physical insecurities. Choose the most unexpected moments. Whisper something like how hot her butt looks in those jeans while you're in a queue at the grocery store.

"I like the way you... ahhh."

That's right. Sometimes, it's best not to finish the sentence at all. This trick works by playing to your lover's emotions. And we all know that the fastest way to get a woman to come (other than hitting her clit, her vaginal walls, and her G-spot simultaneously) is to fuck her feelings. When you're unable to finish your sentence, it makes her feel like your thoughts and emotions are just too intense to put into words. She'll love the fact that she's making you lose your ability to come up with a complete sentence.

"How did you feel when I _____?"

Ex: "How did you feel when I rubbed your clit with my thigh?"

Any questions that you ask during dirty talk must be confident and open-ended. It serves a double purpose. One is to get valuable feedback and the other is to rerun the steamy incident into her memory.

"I'm going to____ ."

Ex: "I'm going to lift your skirt up, pull your panties down, and give you some good spanking.

Make your woman tremble with anticipation by telling her just what you intend to do to her. Women are attracted to men who know how to take control in the bedroom.

"I love it when you ____ ."

Ex: "I love it when you grab the sheets and scream for me to fuck you harder."

When you compliment a woman's actions in bed, it's likely to guarantee a repeat performance. This is a subtle way of telling your lady love just what you want her to do for you without making her feel like you're pressuring her.

Naughty words to say to your man:

"I'm close to coming."

It is important to update your man about your level of arousal. This ensures that you remain on the same page. This works to increase his arousal and it also guides him in adjusting the pace of your lovemaking. Additionally, when you vocalize what's currently going on with your body, this helps bring about awareness.

"Keep doing what you're doing."

Men love it when women give them directions instead of expecting them to read their minds. This is a great way to let your man know that he's on the right path. At the same time, you're indirectly praising his skill thus, motivating him and building his confidence.

"I want you to…"

Ex: "I want you to suck my toes."

"Want" is such a powerful word. It's such a shame that not too many women use it in bed. Men appreciate women who are confident enough to know what they want - and where, when and how they want it.

"I love it when you touch/kiss me... here."

Don't just say it. Grab his hand or guide his mouth towards whichever part of your body you want to be touched or kissed. This trick is effective because it automatically ties up the sexy word with a sexy action.

"You drive me wild when you ____."

Ex: "You drive me wild when you nibble on my clit."

It's a total turn-on for a man when a woman knows exactly what turns her on. But more than that, this phrase is a useful approach for redirecting your man's attention when he's doing something wrong in bed. So rather than saying: "I hate it when you lick my cunt slowly." Use dirty words to reroute his sexual energy towards where you want it the most.

Conclusion

Thank you again for purchasing this book!

I hope this book was able to help you learn how to use the language of lust to improve your sex life and strengthen your relationship.

The next step is to apply these tips in the boudoir and start giving your lover an erotic earful. Have fun being filthy!

Finally, if you enjoyed this book, then I'd like to ask you for a favor; would you be kind enough to leave a review for this book on Amazon? It'd be greatly appreciated! I am a self published author who would need all the help I could get. If you did not like the book, please send me a message at jennifer-amor@gmail.com.

Go to amazon.com to leave a review if you liked the book.

Make sure to check out my other books as well. For example:

Sex: Kama Sutra Sex: Discover the Best Essential Kama Sutra Love Making Techniques to Making Your Lover Addicted to You

(Search for it on amazon)

Now to your FREE gift! I am working with a company which has an email list where you can great offers and info about books on $2.99, $0.99 or FREE promotions.

Do you want to join it? It is 100% free for you if you use the link below and they guarantee that there will be no spam whatsoever. 1-2 emails a week with some book tips, that's it.

(Obs. You have the paperback version. Go to amazon to download the online version of this book for free and get the special link)

Thank you and good luck!

Printed in Great Britain
by Amazon